Fatigue & Fear

12 Daily Practices

By Charles Runels, MD

Find more help at:
www.365HealthStrategies.com

Defeat Fatigue & Fear

Beginning

Here are 12 Practices that
defeat fatigue and fear.

Freedom hides in discipline.

Disregard one of these and risk
being pinned by a bolder of
fatigue, while the poison fog of
fear chokes inspiration from your
chest.

These are not rules to follow.
These are not facts to know.

These are ideas to practice,
Routinely,
Every day.

But, relax—
None practice perfectly.

Just practice.

Practice does not make perfect.

Practice does not make without
fear. Practice makes fear-less.

Defeat Fatigue & Fear

Practice does not make without
sleep. Practice makes tire-less.

You do not defeat fear and
fatigue to know neither—that
would be maniacal.

You defeat fear by blowing away
the poison fog
with the fresh wind of action.

You defeat fatigue by smashing
the bolder
into steps to purpose.

Use the 12 Practices and you will
defeat fatigue and fear—claiming
strength, courage, and direction.

Then, the next day,
practice again.

Charles Runels, MD
May 27, 2014
Still practicing; still not perfect.

Defeat Fatigue & Fear

Notes:

Defeat Fatigue & Fear
12 Daily Practices

1. Rest
2. Fast
3. Play
4. Enjoy
5. Look
6. Sweep
7. Eat
8. Walk
9. Release
10. Ignore
11. Stop
12. Speak

12 Practices to Defeat Fatigue and Fear

Practice 1

Rest.

Claim one day per week of rest. GOD rested. Prophets, thinkers, and happy-healthy people, all rest.

Honeybees do not rest; they work every day. But bees gather mechanically. They work an assembly line, without art, without inspiration.

The GOD in you wants to create the nectar of Love that human bees gather to their hive.

That requires rest.

Rest is not no-thing;
Rest is re-connecting.
Rest is re-creating.

Defeat Fatigue & Fear

Notes:

Practice 2

Fast

Also rest from food:
only water or dilute juice on
your day of rest.

Rest is not no-thing.
Rest is metabolic rebooting.
Rest is mental clearing.

Your Inner Voice and schedule
will tell you which day you
should rest.

Tuesday, Saturday, or Sunday—
you will know which day works
best for you.

Decide the day and keep it
sacred because it is needed—
not needed because it is sacred.

And if someone falls into a ditch
on your day of rest, help him
out.

But, on your day of rest, stay
away from ditches.

Defeat Fatigue & Fear

Notes:

Practice 3

Play.

All animals play. Play is
breathing for something more
than lungs.

Watch the dolphin jump from
the sea. Does she arrive sooner
for going vertical?

Watch the dog that circles
chasing his tail. Do you see the
smile? Only people think
themselves to important to play.

Work without play becomes
uninspired drudgery.
Play without work becomes
vacation from nothing.

If work becomes drudgery, play.
If play becomes boredom, work.

Every day—work.
Every day—play.

Then rest.

Defeat Fatigue & Fear

Notes:

Practice 4

Enjoy.

Enjoy everything. Gratitude
without enjoyment is a lie.
Enjoyment becomes gratitude.

Enjoy your work (which is Love
made concrete) or find new
work. Just decide to enjoy.

Enjoy and find gratefulness for
the water that washes across
your hands and face when you
wake, for the taste of the first
liquid to pass your lips in the
morning, for your lover's kiss, for
your morning prayer, for the air
that passes down the pipe to
your lungs to give you the ability
to think about the morning sky.

Enjoy sorrow. Sorrow is the
vision that allows you to see joy;
the possible sorrow of tomorrow
is the timekeeper that pushes
you to joy and gratitude today.

Defeat Fatigue & Fear

Notes:

Practice 5

Look.

If you direct all your thoughts to
your career, your family, your
self, then you develop tunnel
vision that leads to numbness
and boredom.

Everything relates to everything.
Stop directing all your thoughts
toward yourself; look away from
your private concerns to the
universe outside.

By looking outside yourself, you
awaken to new worlds and new
possibilities and new energy that
you then import back to your
world to make it larger. You also
take what's in your world and
find new ways to contribute to
the universe around you.

Develop and study new interests.
Study literature, dance, marital
arts, music, gardening, science,
or flowers—you decide.

Defeat Fatigue & Fear

Notes:

Practice 6

Sweep.

Sweep your mind of the poisons
that will dull you to an
anesthesia of fatigue and fear.

Take time to write a list of every
worry, every anger,
every resentment,
every prejudice and jealousy.

Then, find an action for each
item. Sweeping is not
forgetting. Sweeping is acting.

Do something toward a solution
for every worry, even if it does
not completely solve the
problem.

Do an act of kindness toward
those for whom you feel poison.

Without regular cleaning, a floor
becomes uninviting to tread.
Without regular sweeping, your
mind becomes uninviting to joy.

Defeat Fatigue & Fear

Notes:

Practice 7

Eat.

Eat at least 5 servings of fresh fruits or vegetables every day.

When you bite the apple with seeds still able to grow a tree, you swallow vitality.

No need to fear food that is not still living, but make sure you daily swallow adequate amounts life.

Except for days of fasting, 5 servings per day (a serving is one cup of vegetables or a medium piece of fruit) is the minimum—more is better.

Water brings life to the seed and water brings life to your body.

Drink 2 liters of water per day.

Defeat Fatigue & Fear

Notes:

Practice 8

Walk.

Walk 3 to 5 miles in the fresh air—every day. A comfortable jog also works.

If safety or severe weather dictates that you walk inside, then use an elliptical trainer and still go the distance. Always, at least walk a short distance in the fresh air every day.

You will find more magic and health than is widely known in the meditation and movement of walking.

On rest days, you can rest from walking.

Add other activities if you wish. But, always walk. Always.

Making 21 miles per week a religion helps make miracles appear in prayer.

Defeat Fatigue & Fear

Notes:

Practice 9

Release.

Release responsibility for results.
Take responsibility for doing
your best effort at work today.

Think, "What is the highest good
that I can do today?"

Then, focus and work.

Work with your head and hands
and not with your emotions.

Let go of the results.

Hold sacred the moment of
practice.

Do not worry that your work
does not seem important. All
things work together. Do not
worry that you may not see the
result you intended.

Use results to redirect work,
then all work is fruitful.

Defeat Fatigue & Fear

Notes:

Practice 10

Ignore.

The only opinion that matters is
your opinion while connected to
GOD. Worrying about the
opinions of others donates your
blood to a ditch.

You will make enemies and
endear lovers with any action—
good or evil, constructive or
destructive.

Ignore the inner doubt that
whispers the sacrilegious,
"What will people think?"

Heeding the sacrilegious, you
will then hear your Inner Voice
call, "Coward," casting you into
darkness.

Ignore outside voices (fan and
critic). Connect only to Timeless
Truth. Then you defeat fear and
fatigue and enjoy energy and
courage.

Defeat Fatigue & Fear

Notes:

Practice 11

Stop.

Whatever you are frantically
doing (thinking that the world
will end if you stop)—stop doing
it.

Stop and number your days and
know that the world will soon
keep going without you.

Though you may think that you
must save your family, your
business, and the world—if you
do not care for your Self, you
cannot.

So, stop.

Prayer, meditation, and
concentration—all words for
something without words.

Stop (even the words)
turn inward and connect
to the source of all doing.

Defeat Fatigue & Fear

Notes:

Defeat Fatigue & Fear

Practice 12

Speak

Speak, out loud,
Words of scripture
And affirmation.

In your beginning is your word.

Speak in songs.
Do not worry about imperfect
rhythm and tune;
Words matter most.

Speak in prose.

Read out loud.

Memorize.
Recite.

Speak and sing inspired words of
strength and courage.

You will defeat fatigue and fear.

Practice.

Now.

Defeat Fatigue & Fear

Notes:

About the Author

Charles Runels, MD did his undergraduate work and received his B.S. degree in chemistry from Birmingham-Southern College. He worked for three years as a product developer and researcher in physics & chemistry at Southern Research Institute designing instrumentation still used by the US armed forces.

He then completed medical school at the University of Alabama in Birmingham, after which he completed his residency and became board-certified in internal medicine.

During 12 years as an ER physician, he founded the largest group of ER physicians in his state while also serving as the medical director of a hyperbaric chamber used for wound care.

He then began a private internal medical practice and conducted clinical trials. He contributed to multiple, peer-reviewed, scientific publications in the areas of hypertension, hormone replacement, and immunology.

In cosmetic medicine, he designed a specific way of using growth factors to rejuvenate the face, commonly called the Vampire Facelift®.

Defeat Fatigue & Fear

His professional organizations include the _Association of Clinical Research Professionals_. He founded the American Cosmetic Cellular Medicine Association (www.ACCMA.memberlodge.org) to help promote further investigation in that area.

His recent work includes research on urinary incontinence and sexual function in both men and women, resulting in his development of the O-Shot® (www.OShot.info) and the Priapus Shot® (www.PriapusShot.com).

Based on his research, he coined the terms and developed the ideas of the "Female Orgasm System" and the "O-Spot" and authored books that include _Activate the Female Orgasm System_ and _Anytime...for as Long as You Want: Strength, Genius, Libido, & Erection by Integrative Sex Transmutation_ (which ran for three years as the best-selling sex manual on Amazon.com).

He is the father of three sons and lives in Fairhope, Alabama.

Charles Runels, MD
www.Runels.com

Other Writings & Inventions of Dr. Runels

www.365HealthStrategies

www.Runels.com

www.OShot.info

www.PriapusShot.com

www.VampireFacelift.com

www.VampireFacial.com

www.VampireBreastLift.com

www.OrgasmSystem.com

Made in the USA
Columbia, SC
08 November 2022